KIDNEY DISEASE DIET COOKBOOK

By

DR. VICKIE STOCK

KIDNEY DISEASE DIET COOKBOOK

TABLE OF CONTENT

INTRODUCTION 7

    What is a kidney? 7

    Principles Of a Kidney Disease Diet 8

    Functions of the kidney 10

    Causes of kidney Diseases 12

    Types of Kidney Diseases 14

    Symptoms of Kidney Diseases 16

    Benefits of Kidney Disease Diet 18

    Kidney Disease Preventive Measures 20

    Kidney Disease foods to eat and avoid 23

KIDNEY DISEASE RECIPES 26

    Blueberry Oatmeal: 26

    Banana Nut Smoothie: 26

    Vegetable Egg Scramble: 27

    Yogurt Parfait: 28

    Quinoa Breakfast Bowl: 29

    Apple Cinnamon Muffins: 29

Sweet Potato Hash Browns:...................................... 30

Avocado Toast with Poached Eggs: 31

Cottage Cheese Pancakes:... 32

Mixed Berry Smoothie Bowl:..................................... 33

Grilled Chicken Salad:.. 34

Tuna and Avocado Wrap:... 34

Mediterranean Quinoa Salad: 35

Vegetable Lentil Soup:... 36

Grilled Salmon with Lemon Dill Sauce:...................... 37

Stuffed Bell Peppers: 38

Greek Chicken Pita Pocket: 39

Lemon Garlic Shrimp Stir-Fry:................................... 40

Hummus and Vegetable Wrap: 42

Tomato Basil Pasta Salad:.. 43

Baked Lemon Herb Salmon:....................................... 43

Vegetarian Stir-Fry with Tofu:.................................... 44

Grilled Chicken with Rosemary Potatoes:.................... 46

Eggplant Parmesan: 47

Lemon Herb Grilled Shrimp: 48

Spinach and Mushroom Frittata: 49

Sesame Ginger Tofu Stir-Fry: 50

Baked Cod with Herbed Quinoa: 51

Roasted Vegetable Couscous Bowl: 52

Mediterranean Chickpea Salad: 53

Apple Cinnamon Cottage Cheese: 54

Carrot and Hummus Sticks: 55

Greek Yogurt with Berries: 55

Cucumber Avocado Bites: 56

Trail Mix Delight: 56

Rice Cake with Tuna Salad: 57

Edamame and Cherry Tomatoes: 58

Cottage Cheese and Pineapple Cups: 58

Watermelon Feta Bites: 59

Berry Chia Pudding: 60

Baked Apples: 60

Chia Seed Pudding: 61

Frozen Banana Bites: 62

Berry Parfait: 63

Coconut Rice Pudding: 63

Yogurt Fruit Salad: 64

Peanut Butter Banana Bites: 65

Mixed Berries Sorbet: 65

Cinnamon Baked Pears: 66

Watermelon Mint Salad: 67

CONCLUSION 68

INTRODUCTION

What is a kidney?

A kidney is a vital organ in the human body that plays a crucial role in maintaining overall health and well-being. Humans typically have two kidneys, one on each side of the spine, located just below the ribcage. They are bean-shaped and about the size of a fist.

The primary function of the kidneys is to filter the blood, removing waste products, excess fluids, and toxins from the body. This process helps regulate the body's internal balance, including the levels of electrolytes, minerals, and fluid.

The waste and excess substances filtered by the kidneys are then converted into urine, which is eventually excreted from the body.

In addition to waste removal, the kidneys also play essential roles in various bodily functions. They produce hormones that help regulate blood pressure, control red blood cell production, and activate vitamin D for bone health.

Keeping the kidneys healthy is crucial for overall well-being. Certain lifestyle choices, such as maintaining a balanced diet, staying hydrated, and avoiding excessive alcohol and smoking, can contribute to kidney health. Regular medical check-ups and managing underlying health conditions are also essential to prevent kidney diseases and complications.

Principles Of a Kidney Disease Diet

Moderate Protein Intake: Consuming an appropriate amount of protein is essential for overall health, but excessive protein intake can put a strain on the kidneys.

Depending on the stage of kidney disease, healthcare professionals may recommend a moderate protein intake to avoid overburdening the kidneys.

Controlled Sodium Intake: High sodium levels can lead to fluid retention and increased blood pressure, which can be harmful to the kidneys.

Reducing sodium intake by avoiding processed foods, salty snacks, and excessive salt during cooking can help manage blood pressure and fluid balance.

Phosphorus Management: For individuals with advanced kidney disease, it is essential to limit phosphorus intake, as the kidneys may have difficulty removing excess phosphorus from the blood. Foods high in phosphorus, such as dairy products and certain meats, should be consumed in moderation.

Potassium Regulation: People with kidney disease may experience imbalances in potassium levels. Controlling potassium intake by avoiding high-potassium foods, such as bananas, oranges, and tomatoes, can help prevent complications.

Fluid Restriction: In some cases, individuals with kidney disease may be advised to limit fluid intake to prevent fluid overload and swelling.

Balanced Nutrition: A kidney disease diet emphasizes a well-balanced and nutrient-rich approach to eating. It includes a variety of fruits, vegetables, whole grains, lean proteins, and healthy fats to ensure adequate nutrition.

Monitoring Medications: Some medications, such as phosphate binders, may be prescribed to help control phosphorus levels. Adhering to the prescribed medication regimen is essential for managing kidney disease effectively.

Regular Monitoring: Regular check-ups with healthcare professionals are vital to monitor kidney function and adjust the diet and treatment plan as needed.

Functions of the kidney

Filtration of Blood: One of the primary functions of the kidneys is to filter waste products, toxins, and excess substances from the bloodstream. As blood flows through the kidneys, they remove unwanted substances and retain essential nutrients and electrolytes.

Regulation of Fluid Balance: The kidneys play a crucial role in maintaining the body's fluid balance. They adjust the amount of water excreted as urine based on factors such as hydration status and the concentration of substances in the blood.

Electrolyte Balance: The kidneys help regulate the levels of various electrolytes, such as sodium, potassium, calcium, and phosphate, in the bloodstream. Proper electrolyte balance is essential for nerve function, muscle contraction, and overall cellular function.

Blood Pressure Regulation: The kidneys contribute to regulating blood pressure by adjusting the volume of blood and the constriction or dilation of blood vessels. They produce hormones like renin, which play a role in blood pressure control.

Red Blood Cell Production: The kidneys produce a hormone called erythropoietin, which stimulates the bone marrow to produce red blood cells. This hormone is crucial for maintaining a healthy supply of oxygen-carrying red blood cells in the bloodstream.

Acid-Base Balance: The kidneys help maintain the body's acid-base balance by excreting hydrogen ions and retaining bicarbonate ions. This process is vital for maintaining the body's pH level within a narrow range.

Metabolism of Vitamin D: The kidneys are involved in the activation of vitamin D, which is essential for the absorption of calcium and phosphorus from the intestines. Proper vitamin D metabolism supports bone health and overall mineral balance.

Excretion of Metabolic Waste: The kidneys remove metabolic waste products, such as urea and creatinine, from the bloodstream. These waste products are then excreted as urine.

Causes of kidney Diseases

Diabetes: Diabetes is one of the leading causes of kidney disease. High blood sugar levels can damage the blood vessels in the kidneys, impairing their ability to function properly.

High Blood Pressure: Uncontrolled high blood pressure (hypertension) can put strain on the blood vessels in the kidneys, leading to kidney damage over time.

Kidney Infections: Infections in the kidneys, such as pyelonephritis, can cause inflammation and damage to the kidney tissues.

Urinary Tract Obstruction: Blockages in the urinary tract, such as kidney stones or an enlarged prostate, can obstruct the flow of urine and lead to kidney damage.

Glomerulonephritis: Glomerulonephritis is a group of kidney diseases that result from inflammation of the glomeruli, the tiny filtering units in the kidneys.

Polycystic Kidney Disease (PKD): PKD is an inherited condition characterized by the growth of fluid-filled cysts in the kidneys, which can eventually lead to kidney failure.

Autoimmune Disorders: Certain autoimmune diseases, such as lupus and IgA nephropathy, can cause the immune system to attack the kidneys, leading to kidney damage.

Drug Overuse: Prolonged use of certain medications, such as nonsteroidal anti-inflammatory drugs (NSAIDs) and some antibiotics, can cause kidney damage.

Toxic Exposure: Exposure to certain toxins, heavy metals, and chemicals can damage the kidneys and impair their function.

Genetic Factors: Some kidney diseases, such as Alport syndrome and Fabry disease, are caused by genetic mutations that affect the structure and function of the kidneys.

Systemic Diseases: Diseases that affect multiple organs, such as systemic lupus erythematosus (SLE) or vasculitis, can also impact the kidneys.

Age and Aging: As people age, the risk of kidney diseases increases due to natural wear and tear on the kidneys over time.

Types of Kidney Diseases

Chronic Kidney Disease (CKD): CKD is a progressive condition where the kidneys gradually lose their ability to filter waste and excess fluids from the blood. It is often caused by conditions like diabetes and high blood pressure.

Acute Kidney Injury (AKI): AKI is a sudden and severe decline in kidney function, usually caused by a sudden reduction in blood flow to the kidneys or direct kidney damage from infections, toxins, or medications.

Glomerulonephritis: Glomerulonephritis is a group of kidney diseases that involve inflammation of the glomeruli, the filtering units in the kidneys. It can be caused by infections, immune system disorders, or other underlying conditions.

Polycystic Kidney Disease (PKD): PKD is a genetic disorder characterized by the growth of fluid-filled cysts in the kidneys, which can lead to kidney enlargement and impair kidney function over time.

Kidney Stones: Kidney stones are hard mineral and salt deposits that form in the kidneys. They can cause intense pain and block the flow of urine.

Urinary Tract Infections (UTIs): UTIs can lead to kidney infections (pyelonephritis), which can cause kidney damage if left untreated.

Nephrotic Syndrome: Nephrotic syndrome is a condition characterized by large amounts of protein in the urine, low blood protein levels, high cholesterol levels, and swelling (edema).

Hemolytic Uremic Syndrome (HUS): HUS is a rare but serious condition that can lead to kidney failure, often triggered by certain types of bacteria, such as E. coli.

Diabetic Nephropathy: Diabetic nephropathy is a type of kidney damage caused by diabetes. It is one of the leading causes of kidney failure.

IgA Nephropathy: IgA nephropathy is a kidney disease caused by the buildup of the antibody immunoglobulin A (IgA) in the kidneys, leading to inflammation and damage.

Lupus Nephritis: Lupus nephritis is kidney inflammation caused by systemic lupus erythematosus (SLE), an autoimmune disease.

Alport Syndrome: Alport syndrome is a genetic disorder that affects the glomeruli in the kidneys, leading to kidney damage and hearing loss.

Symptoms of Kidney Diseases

Changes in Urination: Changes in urination patterns can be early signs of kidney problems. This may include:

- Frequent urination
- Decreased urine output
- Dark-colored urine
- Foamy or bubbly urine
- Blood in the urine

Swelling (Edema): Kidney diseases can lead to fluid retention, causing swelling in the legs, ankles, feet, and hands.

Fatigue and Weakness: Kidney diseases can result in anemia, a condition where there is a shortage of red blood cells, leading to fatigue and weakness.

Shortness of Breath: As kidney function declines, excess fluid and waste products can build up in the body, leading to shortness of breath.

High Blood Pressure: Kidney diseases can cause or exacerbate high blood pressure, which can further damage the kidneys.

Nausea and Vomiting: Accumulation of waste products in the blood can lead to nausea and vomiting.

Loss of Appetite: Decreased kidney function can cause a loss of appetite and weight loss.

Muscle Cramps: Electrolyte imbalances in the blood, such as low calcium and potassium levels, can cause muscle cramps.

Itching: The buildup of waste products in the blood can cause skin itching.

Sleep Problems: Kidney diseases can disrupt sleep patterns, leading to insomnia or restless legs syndrome.

Puffiness around the Eyes: Swelling around the eyes, especially in the morning, can be a sign of kidney problems.

Metallic Taste in the Mouth: An accumulation of waste products in the blood can lead to a metallic taste or ammonia breath.

Benefits of Kidney Disease Diet

Improved Kidney Function: A kidney disease diet helps reduce the workload on the kidneys by limiting the intake of certain nutrients, such as protein, sodium, potassium, and phosphorus. This can slow the progression of kidney disease and potentially improve kidney function.

Blood Pressure Control: By reducing sodium intake and promoting a balanced diet, a kidney disease diet can help manage high blood pressure, a common complication of kidney disease. Controlling blood pressure is vital for preserving kidney health and preventing further damage.

Fluid Balance: A kidney disease diet may include fluid restrictions for individuals with advanced kidney disease or fluid retention issues. Proper fluid management helps prevent edema and maintains a healthy fluid balance in the body.

Phosphorus Control: For individuals with impaired kidney function, excessive phosphorus intake can be harmful. A kidney disease diet focuses on limiting phosphorus-rich foods, which helps prevent complications related to elevated phosphorus levels.

Potassium Regulation: Maintaining proper potassium levels is crucial for heart and muscle function. A kidney disease diet provides guidelines for managing potassium intake, especially for individuals at risk of high potassium levels.

Proper Nutrition: Despite dietary restrictions, a kidney disease diet emphasizes the importance of consuming adequate nutrition. It includes a variety of nutrient-rich foods to ensure essential vitamins, minerals, and energy are provided.

Prevention of Complications: By managing key nutrients and avoiding foods that can exacerbate kidney problems, a kidney disease diet helps reduce the risk of complications such as electrolyte imbalances, bone disease, and cardiovascular issues.

Improved Quality of Life: Adhering to a kidney disease diet can lead to improved overall health, reduced symptoms, and increased energy levels, leading to a better quality of life for individuals with kidney disease.

Customization: A kidney disease diet can be tailored to the individual's specific condition, stage of kidney disease, and other health considerations, making it a personalized approach to managing kidney health.

Support for Medical Treatment: A well-balanced kidney disease diet complements medical treatments, medications, and other therapies prescribed by healthcare professionals, enhancing the effectiveness of the overall treatment plan.

Kidney Disease Preventive Measures

Maintain a Healthy Blood Pressure: High blood pressure is a leading cause of kidney disease. Regularly monitor your blood pressure and work with your healthcare provider to keep it within a healthy range through lifestyle changes and, if necessary, medication.

Manage Blood Sugar Levels: For individuals with diabetes, keeping blood sugar levels under control is essential. Proper diabetes management can help prevent or delay the onset of diabetic nephropathy, a common kidney disease related to diabetes.

Stay Hydrated: Drinking an adequate amount of water is essential for kidney health.

Proper hydration helps flush out toxins and waste products from the kidneys. However, individuals with kidney disease may require fluid restrictions, so it's essential to follow healthcare provider's recommendations.

Adopt a Balanced Diet: Follow a kidney-friendly diet that is low in sodium, phosphorus, and potassium, and moderate in protein. Focus on fresh fruits, vegetables, whole grains, and lean sources of protein. Avoid processed and high-sodium foods.

Exercise Regularly: Engaging in regular physical activity can help maintain a healthy weight, control blood pressure, and improve overall cardiovascular health, which is beneficial for kidney function.

Limit Alcohol Consumption: Excessive alcohol intake can strain the kidneys and increase the risk of kidney damage. Limit alcohol consumption to moderate levels or as advised by a healthcare provider.

Quit Smoking: Smoking can damage blood vessels and reduce kidney function. Quitting smoking is essential for overall kidney and cardiovascular health.

Monitor Medications: Some medications, including over-the-counter pain relievers and certain prescription drugs, can harm the kidneys when used long-term or in excessive doses. Always follow dosing instructions and consult a healthcare provider before taking new medications.

Avoid Nephrotoxic Substances: Be cautious about exposure to toxins and chemicals that can harm the kidneys, such as certain drugs, solvents, and heavy metals.

Regular Health Check-ups: Schedule regular health check-ups with your healthcare provider. Routine screening can detect kidney problems early, enabling timely intervention and management.

Manage Underlying Conditions: If you have conditions like diabetes, high blood pressure, or autoimmune disorders, work closely with your healthcare provider to manage these conditions effectively and reduce their impact on kidney health.

Avoid Self-Medication: Avoid self-prescribing medications, supplements, or herbal remedies without consulting a healthcare provider, as some of these substances can be harmful to the kidneys.

Kidney Disease foods to eat and avoid

Fresh Fruits: Apples, berries, cherries, grapes, peaches, and pears are generally kidney-friendly due to their lower potassium content.

Vegetables: Asparagus, cauliflower, cucumber, eggplant, green beans, lettuce, onions, and bell peppers are lower in potassium and suitable for kidney health.

White Bread and Rice: These alternatives are lower in phosphorus compared to whole wheat and brown rice.

Lean Proteins: Choose skinless chicken, turkey, fish, and egg whites as they are lower in phosphorus and potassium. Small portions of lean beef or pork may also be included.

Dairy Alternatives: Opt for dairy substitutes like almond milk, rice milk, or coconut milk, which are lower in phosphorus.

Olive Oil: Use olive oil or other healthy oils instead of butter or lard to reduce saturated fat intake.

Egg Whites: Egg whites are a protein source with minimal phosphorus and potassium compared to whole eggs.

Herbs and Spices: Flavor foods with herbs and spices like garlic, oregano, basil, and thyme, rather than using salt.

Cabbage: Cabbage can be beneficial for kidney health as it is low in potassium.

- **Foods to Avoid (High-Potassium and High-Phosphorus Foods):**

Bananas: Bananas are high in potassium and should be limited in a kidney-friendly diet.

Oranges and Orange Juice: These are high in potassium and should be consumed in moderation.

Tomatoes and Tomato Products: Tomato-based products, including sauces and ketchup, are high in potassium.

Potatoes and Sweet Potatoes: These are rich in potassium and should be limited in the diet.

Dried Fruits: Raisins, prunes, and other dried fruits are high in potassium and phosphorus.

Processed Meats: Deli meats, bacon, and sausages are high in sodium and should be avoided or limited.

High-Phosphorus Foods: Avoid high-phosphorus foods like chocolate, nuts, seeds, and colas.

Pickled Foods: Pickles and pickled vegetables are high in sodium and should be limited.

Canned Foods: Canned soups, vegetables, and beans are high in sodium and should be avoided or chosen with no added salt options.

Processed Snacks: Chips, pretzels, and crackers are typically high in sodium and should be limited.

KIDNEY DISEASE RECIPES

Blueberry Oatmeal:

Ingredients:

½ cup rolled oats

1 cup water

½ cup blueberries

1 tablespoon honey (optional)

Instructions:

In a saucepan, bring water to a boil.

Add rolled oats and cook on low heat for 5 minutes, stirring occasionally.

Once oats are cooked, stir in blueberries and honey (if using).

Serve hot.

Banana Nut Smoothie:

Ingredients:

1 ripe banana

1 cup unsweetened almond milk

2 tablespoons chopped walnuts

1 teaspoon honey (optional)

Instructions:

In a blender, combine banana, almond milk, and walnuts.

Blend until smooth.

Add honey for sweetness (if desired) and blend again.

Pour into a glass and enjoy.

Vegetable Egg Scramble:

Ingredients:

2 eggs

1 tablespoon chopped bell peppers

1 tablespoon chopped onions

1 tablespoon chopped spinach

1 teaspoon olive oil

Instructions:

In a bowl, whisk the eggs until well combined.

Heat olive oil in a non-stick pan over medium heat.

Add chopped vegetables and sauté for 2-3 minutes.

Pour the whisked eggs into the pan and scramble until cooked through.

Serve hot.

Yogurt Parfait:

Ingredients:

1 cup plain Greek yogurt

½ cup sliced strawberries

2 tablespoons granola (low-sugar)

1 teaspoon honey (optional)

Instructions:

In a glass or bowl, layer Greek yogurt, sliced strawberries, and granola.

Drizzle honey over the top (if desired).

Repeat the layers.

Enjoy this refreshing parfait.

Quinoa Breakfast Bowl:

Ingredients:

½ cup cooked quinoa

¼ cup low-fat milk

1 tablespoon chopped almonds

1 tablespoon dried cranberries

Instructions:

In a bowl, mix cooked quinoa and milk.

Top with chopped almonds and dried cranberries.

Heat in the microwave for 1-minute or enjoy cold.

Apple Cinnamon Muffins:

Ingredients:

1 cup almond flour

1 teaspoon baking powder

½ teaspoon cinnamon

1 large apple, grated

2 eggs

¼ cup unsweetened applesauce

Instructions:

Preheat the oven to 350°F (175°C) and line a muffin tin with paper liners.

In a bowl, mix almond flour, baking powder, and cinnamon.

Add grated apple, eggs, and applesauce, and stir until well combined.

Spoon the batter into the muffin tin.

Bake for 15-20 minutes or until a toothpick inserted comes out clean.

Let the muffins cool before serving.

Sweet Potato Hash Browns:

Ingredients:

1 medium sweet potato, grated

1 tablespoon olive oil

½ teaspoon paprika

Salt and pepper to taste

Instructions:

Heat olive oil in a non-stick pan over medium heat.

Add grated sweet potato and sauté until tender.

Season with paprika, salt, and pepper.

Cook until the edges are crispy.

Serve as a nutritious side dish.

Avocado Toast with Poached Eggs:

Ingredients:

2 slices whole-grain bread

1 ripe avocado

2 large eggs

Salt and pepper to taste

Instructions:

Toast the whole-grain bread slices.

Mash the ripe avocado and spread it evenly on the toast.

Poach the eggs in boiling water until desired doneness.

Place the poached eggs on top of the avocado toast.

Season with salt and pepper.

Serve warm.

Cottage Cheese Pancakes:

Ingredients:

1 cup low-fat cottage cheese

2 large eggs

½ cup oat flour

1 teaspoon vanilla extract

Instructions:

In a blender, combine cottage cheese, eggs, oat flour, and vanilla extract.

Blend until smooth.

Heat a non-stick pan over medium heat and coat with cooking spray.

Pour the pancake batter onto the pan to form small pancakes.

Cook until bubbles appear on the surface, then flip and cook the other side.

Serve with fresh fruits or a drizzle of honey.

Mixed Berry Smoothie Bowl:

Ingredients:

1 cup frozen mixed berries (blueberries, strawberries, raspberries)

½ cup unsweetened almond milk

1 tablespoon chia seeds

Fresh berries for topping

Instructions:

In a blender, blend frozen mixed berries and almond milk until smooth.

Pour the smoothie into a bowl.

Sprinkle chia seeds on top and add fresh berries for garnish.

Enjoy with a spoon.

Grilled Chicken Salad:

Ingredients:

4 ounces grilled chicken breast, sliced

2 cups mixed salad greens

½ cup cherry tomatoes, halved

¼ cup sliced cucumber

2 tablespoons balsamic vinaigrette dressing (low-sodium)

Instructions:

In a large bowl, combine salad greens, cherry tomatoes, and sliced cucumber.

Top with grilled chicken slices.

Drizzle the balsamic vinaigrette dressing over the salad.

Toss gently and serve.

Tuna and Avocado Wrap:

Ingredients:

4 ounces canned tuna (packed in water), drained

1 small ripe avocado, mashed

2 whole-grain tortillas

½ cup baby spinach leaves

Instructions:

In a bowl, mix drained tuna with mashed avocado.

Lay the tortillas flat and place baby spinach leaves in the center.

Spread the tuna and avocado mixture over the spinach.

Roll up the tortillas into wraps and cut in half.

Enjoy this protein-rich lunch option.

Mediterranean Quinoa Salad:

Ingredients:

1 cup cooked quinoa

½ cup diced cucumber

½ cup halved cherry tomatoes

¼ cup crumbled feta cheese

2 tablespoons chopped Kalamata olives

2 tablespoons chopped fresh parsley

2 tablespoons lemon juice

1 tablespoon olive oil

Instructions:

In a large bowl, combine cooked quinoa, cucumber, cherry tomatoes, feta cheese, and olives.

In a small bowl, whisk together lemon juice and olive oil.

Drizzle the dressing over the quinoa salad and toss to combine.

Garnish with chopped fresh parsley before serving.

Vegetable Lentil Soup:

Ingredients:

1 cup red lentils, rinsed and drained

1 cup chopped carrots

1 cup chopped celery

1 cup chopped zucchini

4 cups low-sodium vegetable broth

1 teaspoon dried thyme

Salt and pepper to taste

Instructions:

In a large pot, combine red lentils, chopped carrots, celery, and zucchini.

Add vegetable broth and bring to a boil.

Reduce heat and simmer for 20-25 minutes or until lentils and vegetables are tender.

Stir in dried thyme, salt, and pepper.

Serve this nutritious soup warm.

Grilled Salmon with Lemon Dill Sauce:

Ingredients:

2 4-ounce salmon fillets

1 tablespoon olive oil

1 tablespoon fresh lemon juice

1 teaspoon dried dill weed

Salt and pepper to taste

Instructions:

Preheat the grill to medium-high heat.

In a small bowl, mix olive oil, lemon juice, dried dill weed, salt, and pepper.

Brush the salmon fillets with the olive oil mixture.

Grill the salmon for 4-5 minutes per side or until fully cooked.

Serve with a side of steamed vegetables.

Stuffed Bell Peppers:

Ingredients:

2 large bell peppers (red or green)

1 cup cooked quinoa

½ cup diced tomatoes

½ cup cooked ground turkey or chicken

¼ cup diced onions

1 clove garlic, minced

1 teaspoon olive oil

1 teaspoon dried oregano

Salt and pepper to taste

Instructions:

Preheat the oven to 375°F (190°C).

Cut the tops off the bell peppers and remove the seeds.

In a skillet, heat olive oil over medium heat.

Sauté onions and garlic until fragrant and tender.

Add cooked ground turkey or chicken, diced tomatoes, dried oregano, salt, and pepper. Cook until heated through.

Stir in cooked quinoa and mix well.

Stuff the bell peppers with the quinoa mixture.

Place the stuffed peppers in a baking dish and bake for 20-25 minutes or until peppers are tender.

Serve hot.

Greek Chicken Pita Pocket:

Ingredients:

4 ounces grilled chicken breast, sliced

2 whole-grain pita bread pockets

½ cup diced cucumbers

½ cup diced tomatoes

¼ cup crumbled feta cheese

2 tablespoons Greek yogurt

1 tablespoon chopped fresh dill

Instructions:

Cut the whole-grain pita bread pockets in half to form pockets.

In a small bowl, mix Greek yogurt with chopped fresh dill.

Stuff each pita pocket with sliced grilled chicken, diced cucumbers, diced tomatoes, and crumbled feta cheese.

Drizzle the Greek yogurt dill sauce over the fillings.

Serve as a delicious and portable lunch option.

Lemon Garlic Shrimp Stir-Fry:

Ingredients:

8 ounces peeled and deveined shrimp

1 cup sliced bell peppers (assorted colors)

1 cup broccoli florets

2 tablespoons olive oil

2 cloves garlic, minced

Zest of 1 lemon

2 tablespoons lemon juice

Salt and pepper to taste

Instructions:

In a large skillet, heat olive oil over medium heat.

Add minced garlic and sauté until fragrant.

Add shrimp to the skillet and cook until they turn pink and opaque.

Stir in sliced bell peppers and broccoli florets, cooking until they are tender-crisp.

Add lemon zest and lemon juice to the stir-fry.

Season with salt and pepper to taste.

Serve this flavorful shrimp stir-fry over cooked quinoa or brown rice.

Hummus and Vegetable Wrap:

Ingredients:

2 whole-grain tortillas

½ cup hummus

1 cup mixed salad greens

½ cup sliced cucumber

½ cup shredded carrots

¼ cup sliced red onion

Instructions:

Lay the whole-grain tortillas flat.

Spread hummus evenly over each tortilla.

Arrange mixed salad greens, sliced cucumber, shredded carrots, and sliced red onion in the center of each tortilla.

Roll up the tortillas into wraps and cut in half.

Enjoy this nutritious and fiber-rich lunch.

Tomato Basil Pasta Salad:

Ingredients:

1 cup cooked whole-grain pasta (penne or fusilli)

1 cup cherry tomatoes, halved

¼ cup chopped fresh basil leaves

2 tablespoons balsamic vinaigrette dressing (low-sodium)

2 tablespoons crumbled feta cheese

Instructions:

In a large bowl, combine cooked pasta, cherry tomatoes, and chopped basil leaves.

Drizzle the balsamic vinaigrette dressing over the pasta salad.

Toss to mix all the ingredients together.

Sprinkle crumbled feta cheese on top before serving.

Baked Lemon Herb Salmon:

Ingredients:

2 salmon fillets

1 tablespoon olive oil

1 tablespoon fresh lemon juice

1 teaspoon dried herbs (such as thyme, oregano, or dill)

Salt and pepper to taste

Instructions:

Preheat the oven to 375°F (190°C).

Place the salmon fillets on a baking sheet lined with parchment paper.

In a small bowl, mix olive oil, lemon juice, dried herbs, salt, and pepper.

Brush the olive oil mixture over the salmon fillets.

Bake in the preheated oven for 15-20 minutes or until the salmon is cooked through.

Serve with steamed vegetables on the side.

Vegetarian Stir-Fry with Tofu:

Ingredients:

1 cup cubed tofu

2 cups mixed stir-fry vegetables (broccoli, bell peppers, snap peas, carrots, etc.)

2 tablespoons low-sodium soy sauce

1 tablespoon sesame oil

1 teaspoon minced garlic

Instructions:

In a large skillet or wok, heat sesame oil over medium-high heat.

Add minced garlic and sauté for a minute.

Add cubed tofu to the skillet and cook until lightly browned.

Stir in mixed stir-fry vegetables and cook until they are tender-crisp.

Pour low-sodium soy sauce over the stir-fry and mix well.

Serve over cooked brown rice or quinoa.

Grilled Chicken with Rosemary Potatoes:

Ingredients:

2 boneless, skinless chicken breasts

2 cups baby potatoes, halved

1 tablespoon olive oil

1 teaspoon dried rosemary

Salt and pepper to taste

Instructions:

Preheat the grill to medium-high heat.

Season chicken breasts with salt and pepper.

Grill the chicken for 5-7 minutes per side or until fully cooked.

In a separate bowl, toss halved baby potatoes with olive oil and dried rosemary.

Grill the potatoes in a vegetable basket for 15-20 minutes or until tender.

Serve grilled chicken with a side of rosemary potatoes.

Eggplant Parmesan:

Ingredients:

1 large eggplant, sliced into rounds

1 cup low-sodium marinara sauce

1 cup shredded mozzarella cheese

¼ cup grated Parmesan cheese

1 tablespoon olive oil

1 teaspoon dried basil

Salt and pepper to taste

Instructions:

Preheat the oven to 375°F (190°C).

Brush eggplant slices with olive oil and season with dried basil, salt, and pepper.

In a baking dish, layer eggplant slices, marinara sauce, and shredded mozzarella cheese.

Repeat the layers and top with grated Parmesan cheese.

Bake in the preheated oven for 25-30 minutes or until the cheese is bubbly and golden.

Serve with a side of mixed greens salad.

Lemon Herb Grilled Shrimp:

Ingredients:

8 ounces peeled and deveined shrimp

1 tablespoon olive oil

1 tablespoon fresh lemon juice

1 teaspoon dried herbs (such as thyme, parsley, or rosemary)

Salt and pepper to taste

Instructions:

In a bowl, whisk together olive oil, lemon juice, dried herbs, salt, and pepper.

Add shrimp to the bowl and toss to coat them with the marinade.

Preheat the grill to medium-high heat.

Thread shrimp onto skewers and grill for 2-3 minutes per side or until they are pink and opaque.

Serve these flavorful grilled shrimp with steamed asparagus.

Spinach and Mushroom Frittata:

Ingredients:

6 large eggs

1 cup chopped fresh spinach

½ cup sliced mushrooms

¼ cup diced onions

½ cup shredded mozzarella cheese

1 tablespoon olive oil

1 teaspoon dried thyme

Salt and pepper to taste

Instructions:

Preheat the oven to 375°F (190°C).

In a large oven-safe skillet, heat olive oil over medium heat.

Sauté diced onions and sliced mushrooms until they are tender.

Add chopped spinach to the skillet and cook until wilted.

In a bowl, whisk together eggs, dried thyme, salt, and pepper.

Pour the egg mixture over the sautéed vegetables in the skillet.

Sprinkle shredded mozzarella cheese on top.

Transfer the skillet to the preheated oven and bake for 15-20 minutes or until the frittata is set.

Serve this protein-packed frittata with a side of mixed green salad.

Sesame Ginger Tofu Stir-Fry:

Ingredients:

1 cup cubed tofu

2 cups mixed stir-fry vegetables (broccoli, snap peas, bell peppers, carrots, etc.)

2 tablespoons low-sodium soy sauce

1 tablespoon sesame oil

1 tablespoon grated fresh ginger

2 cloves garlic, minced

Instructions:

In a large skillet or wok, heat sesame oil over medium-high heat.

Add grated fresh ginger and minced garlic, and sauté for a minute.

Add cubed tofu to the skillet and cook until lightly browned.

Stir in mixed stir-fry vegetables and cook until they are tender-crisp.

Pour low-sodium soy sauce over the stir-fry and mix well.

Serve over cooked brown rice.

Baked Cod with Herbed Quinoa:

Ingredients:

2 4-ounce cod fillets

1 cup cooked quinoa

1 tablespoon olive oil

1 tablespoon fresh lemon juice

1 teaspoon dried herbs (such as thyme, rosemary, or parsley)

Salt and pepper to taste

Instructions:

Preheat the oven to 375°F (190°C).

Place the cod fillets on a baking sheet lined with parchment paper.

In a small bowl, mix olive oil, lemon juice, dried herbs, salt, and pepper.

Brush the olive oil mixture over the cod fillets.

Bake in the preheated oven for 15-20 minutes or until the cod is cooked through.

Serve with herbed quinoa on the side.

Roasted Vegetable Couscous Bowl:

Ingredients:

1 cup cooked whole-wheat couscous

1 cup roasted mixed vegetables (zucchini, bell peppers, cherry tomatoes, etc.)

2 tablespoons balsamic vinaigrette dressing (low-sodium)

1 tablespoon chopped fresh parsley

Instructions:

In a bowl, combine cooked whole-wheat couscous and roasted mixed vegetables.

Drizzle balsamic vinaigrette dressing over the couscous bowl.

Sprinkle chopped fresh parsley on top before serving.

Mediterranean Chickpea Salad:

Ingredients:

1 can (15 ounces) chickpeas, drained and rinsed

1 cup diced cucumbers

1 cup halved cherry tomatoes

½ cup diced red onions

½ cup crumbled feta cheese

2 tablespoons olive oil

2 tablespoons lemon juice

1 teaspoon dried oregano

Salt and pepper to taste

Instructions:

In a large bowl, combine chickpeas, diced cucumbers, halved cherry tomatoes, diced red onions, and crumbled feta cheese.

In a small bowl, whisk together olive oil, lemon juice, dried oregano, salt, and pepper.

Pour the dressing over the chickpea salad and toss to combine.

Serve this refreshing Mediterranean salad as a light and nutritious dinner.

Apple Cinnamon Cottage Cheese:

Ingredients:

1 medium apple, sliced

½ cup low-fat cottage cheese

½ teaspoon ground cinnamon

Instructions:

Arrange apple slices on a plate.

Top with low-fat cottage cheese.

Sprinkle ground cinnamon over the cottage cheese.

Enjoy this protein-packed and fiber-rich snack.

Carrot and Hummus Sticks:

Ingredients:

2 large carrots, cut into sticks

¼ cup hummus (low-sodium)

Instructions:

Place carrot sticks in a serving bowl.

Serve with a side of hummus for dipping.

This snack provides a satisfying crunch and a dose of healthy nutrients.

Greek Yogurt with Berries:

Ingredients:

½ cup plain Greek yogurt (low-fat)

½ cup mixed berries (blueberries, strawberries, raspberries)

Instructions:

In a bowl, spoon plain Greek yogurt.

Top with a mix of fresh berries.

This snack is rich in protein, calcium, and antioxidants.

Cucumber Avocado Bites:

Ingredients:

1 cucumber, sliced into rounds

½ ripe avocado, mashed

1 teaspoon lemon juice

Pinch of salt and pepper

Instructions:

In a small bowl, mix mashed avocado, lemon juice, salt, and pepper.

Place a dollop of avocado mixture on each cucumber round.

These refreshing bites are full of healthy fats and vitamins.

Trail Mix Delight:

Ingredients:

¼ cup unsalted almonds

¼ cup unsalted walnuts

2 tablespoons pumpkin seeds

2 tablespoons dried cranberries

Instructions:

Combine all ingredients in a bowl and mix well.

Portion the trail mix into small snack bags.

This protein-packed snack is perfect for on-the-go.

Rice Cake with Tuna Salad:

Ingredients:

1 rice cake (low-sodium)

½ cup canned tuna, drained and flaked

2 tablespoons Greek yogurt (low-fat)

1 tablespoon chopped celery

1 tablespoon chopped red onion

Salt and pepper to taste

Instructions:

In a bowl, mix canned tuna, Greek yogurt, chopped celery, chopped red onion, salt, and pepper.

Spread the tuna salad over the rice cake.

This light and flavorful snack is high in protein and low in sodium.

Edamame and Cherry Tomatoes:

Ingredients:

1 cup steamed edamame (unsalted)

½ cup cherry tomatoes

Instructions:

Arrange steamed edamame and cherry tomatoes on a plate.

This snack is a great source of plant-based protein and antioxidants.

Cottage Cheese and Pineapple Cups:

Ingredients:

½ cup low-fat cottage cheese

½ cup fresh pineapple chunks

Instructions:

Layer low-fat cottage cheese and fresh pineapple chunks in a serving cup.

This creamy and tropical snack is low in sodium and high in calcium.

Watermelon Feta Bites:

Ingredients:

1 cup watermelon, cut into cubes

2 tablespoons crumbled feta cheese

Fresh mint leaves for garnish

Instructions:

Skewer watermelon cubes and feta cheese on toothpicks.

Garnish with fresh mint leaves.

This refreshing snack is a delightful combination of sweet and savory flavors.

Berry Chia Pudding:

Ingredients:

¼ cup chia seeds

1 cup unsweetened almond milk

½ cup mixed berries (blueberries, raspberries)

1 tablespoon honey (optional)

Instructions:

In a bowl, mix chia seeds and unsweetened almond milk.

Refrigerate the mixture for at least 2 hours or overnight to allow the chia seeds to expand and form a pudding-like consistency.

Before serving, top the chia pudding with mixed berries.

Add honey for sweetness if desired.

This snack is high in fiber and antioxidants.

Baked Apples:

Ingredients:

2 apples, cored and halved

2 tablespoons unsalted butter, melted

1 tablespoon brown sugar substitute

1 teaspoon ground cinnamon

Instructions:

Preheat the oven to 350°F (175°C).

Place the apple halves on a baking sheet.

In a small bowl, mix melted butter, brown sugar substitute, and ground cinnamon.

Brush the mixture over the apple halves.

Bake for 20-25 minutes or until the apples are tender.

Chia Seed Pudding:

Ingredients:

2 tablespoons chia seeds

1 cup unsweetened almond milk

1 tablespoon honey (optional)

½ teaspoon vanilla extract

Instructions:

In a bowl, combine chia seeds, unsweetened almond milk, honey, and vanilla extract.

Stir well and refrigerate for at least 2 hours or overnight to set.

Serve chilled and top with fresh berries if desired.

Frozen Banana Bites:

Ingredients:

2 ripe bananas, sliced

½ cup unsweetened Greek yogurt

2 tablespoons unsweetened cocoa powder

Instructions:

Spread a thin layer of Greek yogurt on one side of each banana slice.

Sandwich two banana slices together, yogurt-side in.

Place the banana bites on a baking sheet lined with parchment paper.

Freeze for 1-2 hours or until firm.

Berry Parfait:

Ingredients:

1 cup low-fat vanilla yogurt

½ cup mixed berries (blueberries, raspberries)

2 tablespoons granola (low-sugar)

Instructions:

In a glass or serving dish, layer low-fat vanilla yogurt, mixed berries, and granola.

Repeat the layers as desired.

This delightful parfait is a great source of vitamins and antioxidants.

Coconut Rice Pudding:

Ingredients:

½ cup cooked white rice

1 cup coconut milk (unsweetened)

1 tablespoon honey (optional)

½ teaspoon vanilla extract

Pinch of ground cinnamon

Instructions:

In a saucepan, combine cooked white rice, coconut milk, honey, vanilla extract, and ground cinnamon.

Simmer over low heat for 10-15 minutes or until the mixture thickens.

Serve warm or chilled.

Yogurt Fruit Salad:

Ingredients:

1 cup diced mixed fruits (pineapple, melon, grapes)

½ cup low-fat plain yogurt

1 tablespoon honey (optional)

1 teaspoon lemon zest

Instructions:

In a bowl, mix diced mixed fruits, low-fat plain yogurt, honey, and lemon zest.

Refrigerate for 10-15 minutes before serving.

Peanut Butter Banana Bites:

Ingredients:

2 ripe bananas, sliced

2 tablespoons unsalted peanut butter

2 tablespoons crushed peanuts (unsalted)

Instructions:

Spread a thin layer of peanut butter on one side of each banana slice.

Sandwich two banana slices together, peanut butter-side in.

Roll the banana bites in crushed peanuts.

Enjoy this protein-packed treat.

Mixed Berries Sorbet:

Ingredients:

2 cups mixed berries (blueberries, strawberries, raspberries)

¼ cup water

1 tablespoon lemon juice

1 tablespoon honey (optional)

Instructions:

In a blender, combine mixed berries, water, lemon juice, and honey.

Blend until smooth.

Pour the mixture into a shallow dish and freeze for 2-3 hours or until firm.

Scoop and serve as a refreshing sorbet.

Cinnamon Baked Pears:

Ingredients:

2 pears, halved and cored

1 tablespoon unsalted butter, melted

1 tablespoon honey (optional)

½ teaspoon ground cinnamon

Instructions:

Preheat the oven to 375°F (190°C).

Place the pear halves on a baking sheet.

In a small bowl, mix melted butter, honey, and ground cinnamon.

Brush the mixture over the pear halves.

Bake for 20-25 minutes or until the pears are tender.

Watermelon Mint Salad:

Ingredients:

2 cups diced watermelon

1 tablespoon fresh mint leaves, chopped

1 tablespoon lime juice

1 teaspoon honey (optional)

Instructions:

In a bowl, combine diced watermelon, chopped fresh mint leaves, lime juice, and honey.

Toss gently to mix.

This light and refreshing dessert is perfect for hot days.

CONCLUSION

adopting a kidney disease diet can be a life-changing and empowering step for individuals with kidney issues. By carefully selecting foods that are kidney-friendly, low in sodium, and rich in essential nutrients, you can significantly improve your kidney health and overall well-being.

This dietary approach aims to manage kidney disease, slow its progression, and alleviate symptoms, ultimately enhancing your quality of life.

The benefits of a kidney disease diet are vast, ranging from better blood pressure control, improved kidney function, and reduced risk of complications like heart disease and kidney failure.

Moreover, by avoiding foods that can strain the kidneys and cause further damage, you are actively taking charge of your health and actively supporting your body's natural healing processes.

However, it's crucial to remember that each person's journey with kidney disease is unique, and consulting with a healthcare professional or a registered dietitian is essential in tailoring a diet plan that best suits your individual needs and medical condition. Regular monitoring, medication adherence, and lifestyle modifications, combined with a kidney-friendly diet, can bring about positive outcomes and pave the way for a healthier future.

By making mindful choices and embracing a kidney disease diet, you are providing your kidneys with the support they need to function optimally, allowing you to live life to the fullest.

Empower yourself with knowledge and take control of your kidney health today—your kidneys will thank you for it, and you can look forward to a brighter and healthier tomorrow. Remember, small changes in your diet can lead to significant improvements in your well-being, one kidney-friendly meal at a time!